3 Hour Window Diet

Glenda L. Maynard

Book cover design concept by Glenda L. Maynard

Library of Congress Cataloging-in-Publication Data is available

Contents

Dedication

I dedicate this book to my three children, my spirit angels.

For Joseph, my youngest, the "Praise & Workout" baby: You were in my womb when I did the job that I loved the most. You heard the beat of every song, and you felt all my dance and workout moves. You are a joy and a pleasure on this earth. Thank you for crashing this party. Training with you is next-level.

For John, my middle child: Memories of our early morning walks and trips to the track are deep in my heart. I remember your encouraging words on the morning run: "you can do it, Mommy!" Thank you also for being the kinder food police in the house. Experimenting with vegetarianism must be one of the marks of the brilliant, intuitive middle child.

For Alyssa, my firstborn and only daughter: Welp, you said that you would read an advice book if I ever wrote one, a memoir, not so much. Ha! I hope you enjoy this advice book (with a small dose of biography). You were my Praise & Workout chief operating officer, hole puncher, record keeper, et al. Your portion controls skills are always on point. You are beautiful on the inside and outside.

I love you three. You are my lights and my purpose.

Foreword

First things first: here are my thoughts on the word "diet."

When selecting the book title, my daughter, who has always been an avid reader, asked if I needed to use the word "diet" in the title. Considering her Gen Z suggestion, I tossed around the idea of NOT using the word "diet."

"Diet" has enough negative connotations and associations as "losing weight" does. Point taken. Back to brainstorming the title.

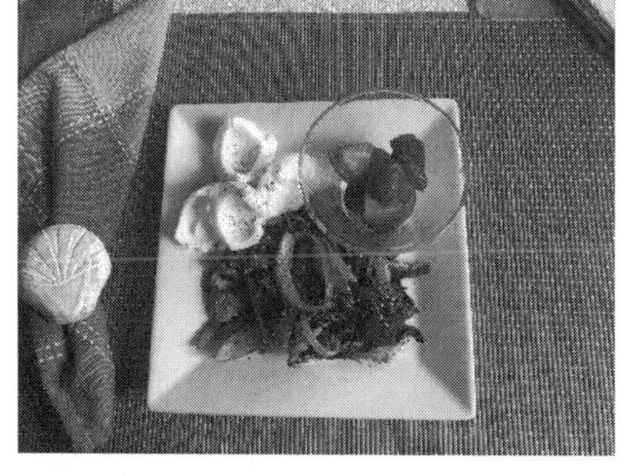

How about "3 Hour Window WOE"? I liked it, and it had a bit of a ring to it.

Only one problem. What is WOE?

In the weight loss community, WOE is an acronym that stands for "way of eating," an ideal way of saying "diet." Your WOE can be OMAD (one meal a day), vegetarian, no carbs, pescatarian, SOFAS free (no salt, oil, flour, alcohol, sugar), the list goes on and on.

Great, but now we have another problem: WOE is a term that is not yet widely used or understood. While I know many may negatively respond to the word "diet," there is no better word in our language that conveys the truth behind what many people need to fix.

3 Hour Window Diet, it is. Enjoy!

Introduction

The who, what, where, when, why and how of *3 Hour Window Diet*

Who is writing this "diet book"?

Yours truly, the author, can teach you how to lose weight because she has lost weight. I am not a medical doctor. I am not a research scientist. Instead, I come to this topic from the perspective of someone who has lost weight, which is significant. Why? Because so many find it nearly "impossible" to "lose weight," even if they are doctors and scientists. As we proceed, I will share more about who I am and why I am the person you should listen to on this topic.

What is the purpose of yet another "diet book," and why is this one special? After all, you already know everything you need to know about how to lose weight.

You know sugar is the devil. You know you have to work out. You know you are supposed to drink water. You know the scale can be your best friend or your worst enemy. You know you are supposed to "shop the perimeters." You know portion control is essential. You know restaurant food is super high in calories, fat, and salt. You know fad diets do not work.

You know all of the above. But have you ever explored the minute by minute, day by day, week by week psychology of food and fitness and how your mind fights you non-stop in the process? Why is this problem such a challenge to solve, given all you know on this topic?

The diet advocated in this book is simple: stop eating so much. At its core, this diet book is about intermittent fasting. Intermittent fasting is not as easy as it seems. I provide tips and tricks to work your way up to more extended periods of fasting and shorter feeding windows.

Ultimately, a 3-hour feeding window executed over several weeks or several months, with breaks in between, will give you the most rapid success. Why is immediate success critical? It's a marathon, not a sprint, correct? Well, sure, in a way. However, we all know that if you see results immediately, you are more inspired to keep going. Action items learned here will carry you into the maintenance phase and enjoyment of this process.

Where the battle is fought and won. Hint: it is not where you think

An ordinary weight loss book would focus your "where" to the kitchen and gym. While I agree "you make your abs in the kitchen," I have also discovered an unlikely place and space to bring the struggle that can get you to another level of awareness and activity if executed in a focused and intentional manner.

In this diet book, the kitchen and the gym are secondary to the cell phone, computer, social media, and old-fashioned pen-to-paper journal. The game-changer activity is not only making up your mind to lose weight but using the power of telling others, posting, and sharing to ensure that your body follows your thoughts and intentions. No one wants friends and loved ones to know that you have not followed through on your stated actions. Here is where bragging and shame intersect. Brag about your intention, then back it up with the effort to avoid SHAME: a powerful equation. Trust me. I promise you it works better than any other "diet plan" that gives you a list of foods, recipes, and meal plans.

When to start and how to beat the procrastination bug

Now. Not next Monday. Not first of the month. Not the first day of the new year. Not when the vernal equinox meets Mars in Jupiter on the full moon of Venus in retrograde. Right. Now. You may not jump to the 3 Hour Window today, day 1, but there is SOMETHING in this book that you can do TODAY. In dieting, adopt this phrase: "there is no such thing as tomorrow." Procrastination ends NOW and TODAY.

Why it is helpful to internalize the concept of "lifelong" journey

Because you keep trying and failing, it is time to try and succeed. Fixing the problem today will help you sustain your effort tomorrow, next month, years from now.

How does *3 Hour Window Diet* work?

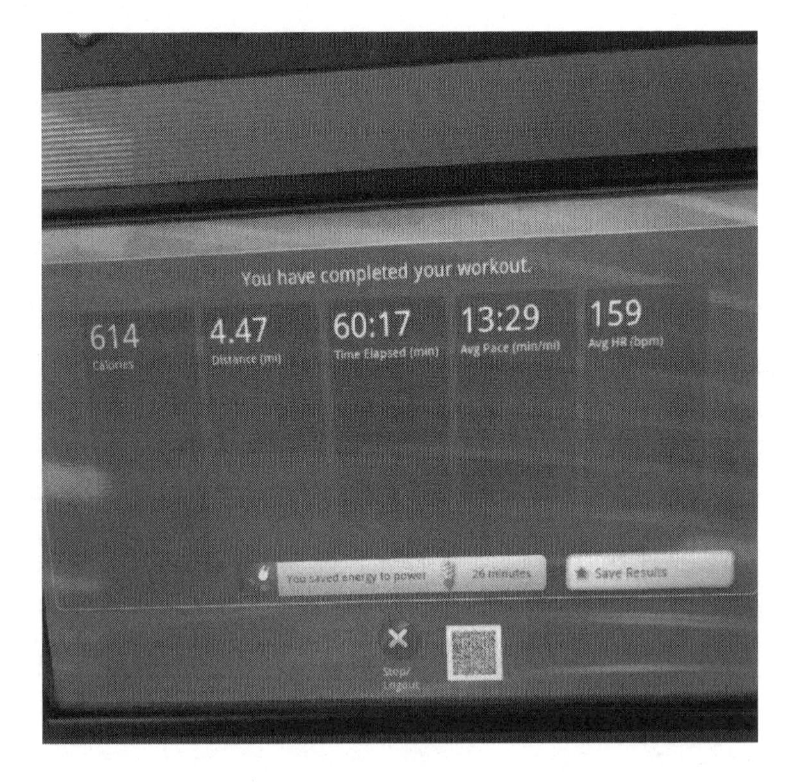

Keep reading and listening.

Snapshot of my weight loss history and body image awareness: 3rd grade - present

If you have never had to lose weight, it is impossible to tell or show someone how to lose weight. Plain. Simple. End of discussion. You may receive some helpful advice from a medical or research perspective, but that community has failed miserably at solving this problem. No offense. They are lost when it comes to fixing how the mind fights the overweight person minute by minute, day by day, week after week, month to month, year to year, over an entire lifetime.

Now that we have gotten that out of the way, let's get into the psyche of a person (like the readers and me) who has had a long-time "obsession" with bodyweight, image, looking great, looking not so great, how it all feels, and how it impacts your choices.

Think back to the first time you remember thinking you were fat. Pause for a moment. Think. Feel that pain.

For me, it was 3rd grade. One of my classmates found a title in the school library called *Me and Fat Glenda* by Lila Perl. Why on earth would someone write a book using my name and calling me fat? Did the author know me? Ugh.

My first name is unusual, one that no other kid in my lifetime of schools shared. Anyone with an uncommon name knows this challenge. A book sat on the library shelf, associating my name with an adjective that everyone understood as ugly and shameful. FAT. Was I a little chubbier than the other kids? Unfortunately, yes.

Once a year, our class took a long walk to the nurses' office, where everyone sat on the floor and waited to hear their name in alphabetical order. Two nurses participated in this cruel event. One nurse would weigh and record the child's height measurement. Then she would call out the dreaded numbers to the other nurse.

Though my height was in the normal range, my weight was probably about 10 pounds higher than most other girls.

Fat. Glenda.

Fast forward to junior year in high school. My prom dress size is a forgotten memory, but I recall weighing about 135 pounds and still thinking of myself as fat, just as in 3rd grade. The cure was to exercise at the gym with my mother; the Stairmaster was her machine of choice. I took group fitness classes and fell in love with step aerobics. Something about "aerobics" in the '80s felt trendy, challenging, and fun.

At the beginning of my senior year in college, I had a party for my 21st birthday, a size eight dress, not sure of my weight. Party night left me feeling comfortable and relatively slim in my skin. To begin the transition into the real world, I moved off-campus and traded the university library circulation job for a gig working front desk at a downtown DC hotel. One of the work perks: our managers permitted us to order a free meal from the hotel restaurant at every shift.

I blamed this extra on-the-job eating for my first experience packing on significant pounds in a relatively short amount of time. "Feeling fat" was not all in my head. I had stopped eating red meat at age 16 and stayed faithful to that cause for five years. Whatever preceded the urge to eat a cheeseburger, there was no turning back as soon as it happened. The hotel's burgers and fries were tasty, and the weight gain betrayed my secretly indulgent lousy habit. By graduation, I had swiftly ballooned up to 176 pounds. A few friends noticed and mentioned it, leaving me to feel self-conscious and guilty. Recently, I showed my daughter a pic from that year. "No, Mommy, you weren't fat! You were thick". Thanks to the body positivity movement, beauty image standards have changed over time, and she did not want me to feel bad. Bless her heart.

After graduation, it was back home to New York and back to the gym. Youth enabled me to drop weight effortlessly, even without following much of a plan. On our wedding day, my weight was average again, perhaps around 140 pounds. Just like prom and 21st birthday party, wedding day showcased a slim and confident Glenda. Fat Glenda was a distant shadow.

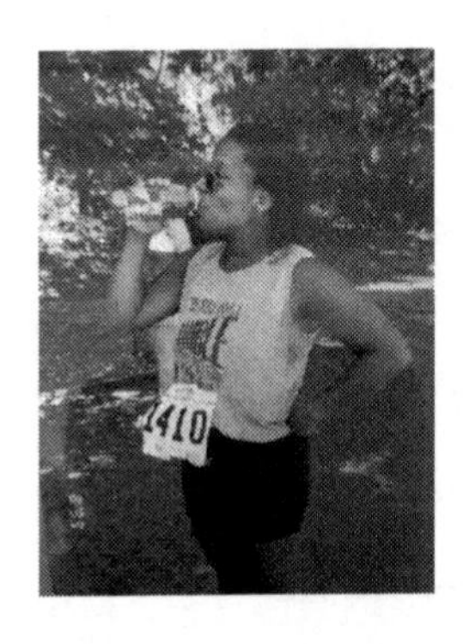

Baby #1. I gained about 20 pounds. Snapback, no problem. After baby #2, an idea bloomed: turn my love of fitness into a business venture. In 2001, my next baby, "Praise & Workout," a church-based fitness program, was born in Bronx, New York.

In the beginning, I taught five classes per week. Best. Shape. Ever. Eating right was natural and effortless for my tight, muscular 150-pound frame. I maintained my dream body for several years and welcomed participants to spend 60 minutes sweating, jumping, dancing, lifting, kicking, punching, and smiling. Praise & Workout was a fully functional side-gig with a logo, website, custom music mixes, radio commercial, and business model that included traveling to other states to share the concept with churches.

Baby #3. Despite concern from a few well-meaning church members, there was no reason to stop teaching until two weeks before the delivery date, with the assistance of a chair and modified movements. Eight weeks after giving birth, I was back at it, albeit a little thicker (163 pounds). Four years of consistently teaching several classes per

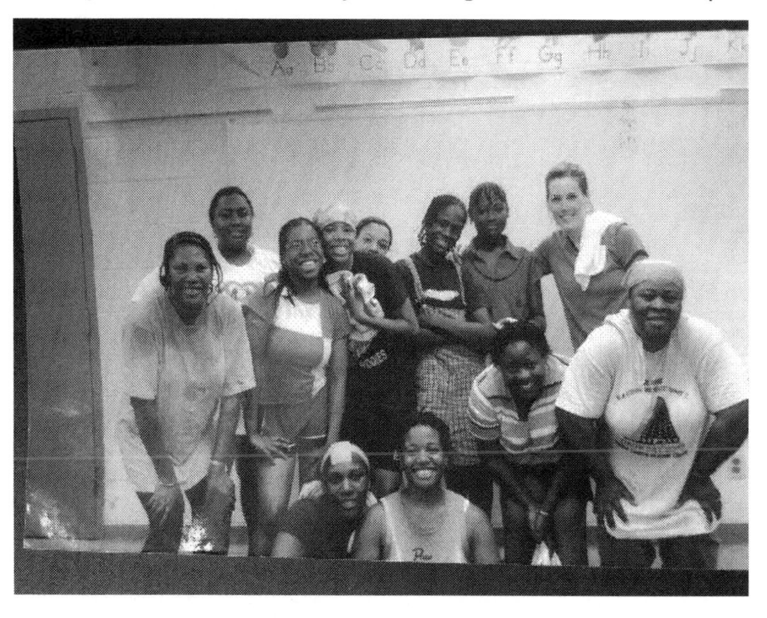

Bottom row, right, sweaty after teaching a class, circa 2003

week helped me feel good, active, and in control of my body. Praise & Workout lived from 2001-2008, sharing heart, body, and soul with over 1000 people. I left my beloved class and participants behind in New York to relocate to another state. Although circumstances dictated a change for me and my children, I was heartbroken to stop teaching fitness and had a profoundly nagging fear that moving and losing my class would cause me to gain weight.

My fear turned out to be unfounded initially. Everything was slightly up and down but mostly fine until 2013 or so. I started to get comfortable in a fundraising job that "required" me to do frequent food-centered entertaining. Free and lavish breakfast, lunch, and dinner events were taking place a few times a week. I piled on weight for three years, not knowing the exact numerical damage, but sure the scale tipped over 200 pounds. That had never been the case for me unless pregnant (only with baby #2 toward the very end). Unpregnant Glenda had no business being 200+ pounds, but there she was. Fat. For real.

During this time, the disturbing part was that I was still working out regularly, albeit not as intensely as when I was teaching back in NY. Walking, treadmill, elliptical, and group fitness were my usual activities. The significant difference, of course, was my diet. I had never so frequently eaten rich and decadent in the past, and it was starting to show on my formerly fit frame. I even signed up for a popular program at work that I am sure you have tried. The program included weekly meetings and weigh-ins. I left each session feeling depressed about the sharing that took place in the group. It made sense that group support would be helpful, but who wanted to feel sad while trying to lose weight? Not me. I think I only lost 5 pounds before I quit.

During these three years, I started to learn everything about what it means to be fat, not imaginary fat in my head, but truly fat in my body. I was not too fond of pictures and scrutinized every image for how fat it made me look or feel. In June 2016, I saw how fat I indeed was when I looked at pictures of me at a cousin's wedding. After posting a pic on Facebook of my dad and me at the wedding, friends still kindly and politely complimented and called me beautiful. Could no one see or feel what I was seeing and feeling? I deleted the picture shortly after posting it, unable to look at the truth.

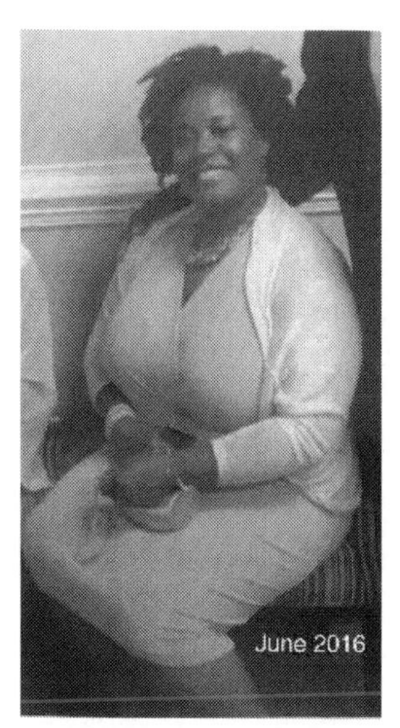
June 2016

Something drastic and different was on the horizon.

In October of 2016, I started a small private group on Facebook called *80/20 Journal*. 80% of why I was gaining weight was my diet. My workouts were only moving the needle 20%, and that was barely enough to stay ahead of all the free and calorie-dense foods I was consuming.

The premise of *80/20 Journal* was a challenge: be honest and open about ALL the food I (and the group) would consume during seven days. Write, take pics, share.

I love that concept of finding a "game-changer," and founding the group certainly qualified as a game-changer for me and others.

This book is based on my 7-year experience as a fitness instructor; and my 4-year experience leading an online accountability group of individuals who all want to achieve the same goal, that elusive "dream body."

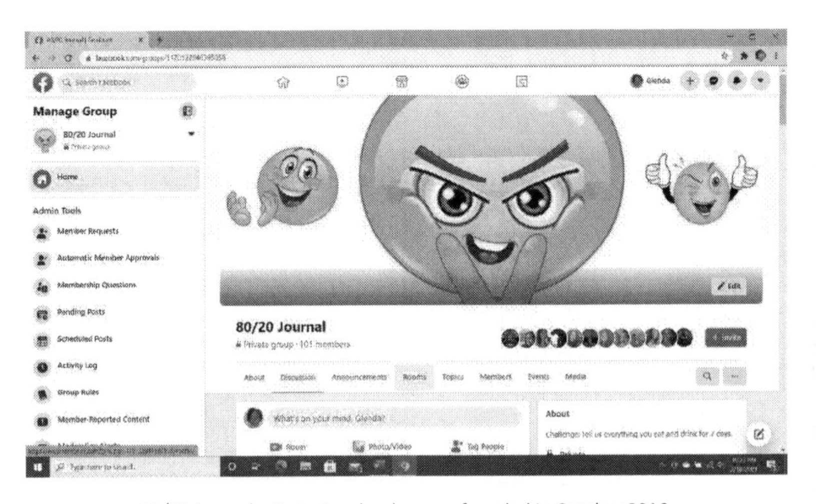

80/20 Journal private Facebook group founded in October 2016

What this diet book is NOT about

This book will not tell you what foods to eat, how to weigh proteins, or which fruits and veggies are the best to blend into a smoothie. This book will not tell you about carb cycling or counting macronutrients. This book will not try to sell you on keto, vegan, or paleo. You know that stuff inside and out. And. Still. Struggle.

Wait.

What kind of diet book is not going to lay out an exact diet for you to FOLLOW?

This kind.

I intend to put YOU in the driver's seat by making YOU in charge of what you put on your plate.

Over the four years of making and reading posts in my private group and observing my behavior, I have learned that the mind is both your friend and your enemy. Minute one: you tell your mind what to do; minute two: your mind starts trying to talk you out of it. When you do what you are not supposed to do, your mind is right there accusing you and telling you to get your act together.

So, what kind of diet book is this?

It is in the title.

This book is about using the clock as a tool for controlling your cravings and food rituals. This book will teach you how to implement behavioral changes and intermittent fasting to crush your body goals in the shortest amount of time possible.

That is the gift we have on this earth: time.

After trying all food combinations, I have discovered that every plan goes out the window when a craving hits or a social invitation pops up. There is a birthday or holiday nearly every month that "requires" you to break diet protocol and eat something you know you should not.

In our food-centered culture, the temptation to eat unnecessarily is lurking every minute of every day.

You already know the list of foods to avoid. We will not focus on that well-known list. Anyone living on this earth knows that pizza and chocolate cake will make you gain weight. I do not have to tell you that, let alone write a whole book about it. Despite everyone knowing the effect of pizza and chocolate cake, we all eat them when we want to. Why is this, and what should we do to minimize pizza and cake's effect on your midsection? This book will help you address

THOSE questions and provide strategies for answering them.

3 Hour Window Diet is a short quick read. Get the information and get on with your fasting day! I encourage you to pick up this book frequently for inspiration and motivation. Working through the end of the book's annual goals will also keep you from losing interest in your "weight loss" along the way. Stagnation is the death of ALL weight loss plans!

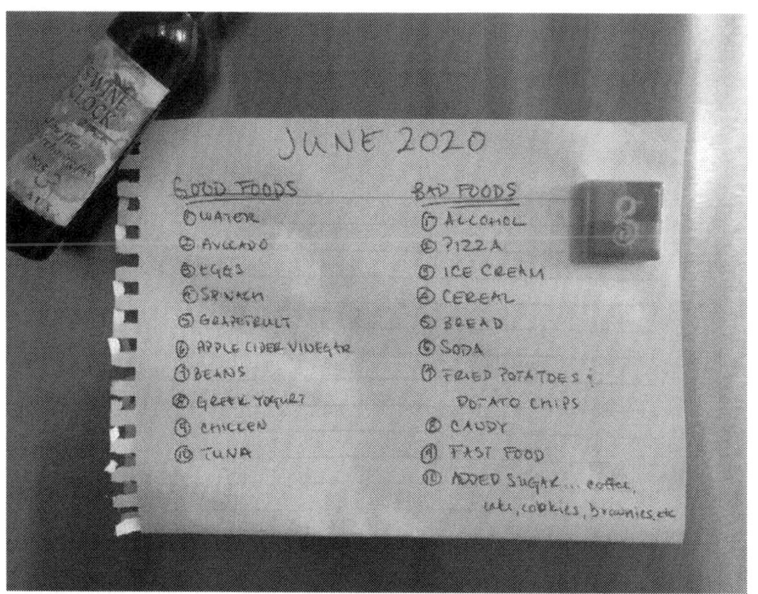

While we are here, I will share something one of our group members posted that lives on my fridge:

There you have it. Just do that list I posted.

Problem solved.

Not so easy, huh? Yup, keep reading.

Bringing the battle to social media

If you are reading or listening to this book, you know the staple "diet" advice. Those of us who have ever attempted to gather information to "lose weight" will have heard several common tips. Here are some examples: Shop the perimeter. Reduce carbs. Eat at least five servings of fruits and veggies daily. Drink half your body weight in ounces of water daily. Blah, blah, blah. I can feel you slipping away from me as you read these stale action items. You are mentally checking out and preparing to resist.

We are going to hit PAUSE on the tried-and-true advice, despite its relative usefulness. Stick a pin in that advice. We will come back to it.

Instead, let's try some different advice.

Prepare. Plate. Snap pic. Post.

What does this mean?

I am suggesting that you change the location of the battlefield to a whole new place. Do not fight cravings in the recesses and privacy of your mind with stale information. Try something different.

By "something different," I mean: Fight the battle in public (well in private) and on social media.

Yes, I said SOCIAL MEDIA.

Wait, what does social media have to do with losing weight?

I will explain it.

When you gain weight, it is usually because you are hiding your food consumption, not because you are "big-boned," "genetically disadvantaged," or "have a thyroid problem." Unless you were diagnosed by a professional, the over-consumption of food directly caused all that personality on your hips. You are ashamed to admit that you secretly eat more and worse than you should. Somehow, your mind tells you that you can get away with eating something, and it is not going to show up on your thighs, or butt, or belly. Your mind is lying to you about many things.

What is the solution to this problem?

Fight your mind with the truth.

If you had to "go public" with everything you ate, trust me, it would automatically force you to behave in a way that hiding and sneaking will not allow. Use shame to correct your bad behavior and replace it with good behavior.

Prepare the healthy foods you already know you are supposed to eat. Plate your meal in a way that is visually appealing and gives honor and respect to the food. Take a picture of your aesthetically appealing, healthy dish. It does not matter that you may feel a little silly doing this. There is a method to the madness. Share the pic with friends or loved ones who know you are struggling with this area of your life.

Enter your new, life-changing, daily habit.

Do not leave the pic on your camera roll. That would be like calling a touchdown at the 40-yard line. Sharing is the critical element.

The moment you feel the compulsion to eat something "inappropriate," you will think twice about eating it.

Let's play it out. Chocolate chip cookies are your weakness if you are anything like me. You are in the grocery store, and the best cookies in the world (you know the ones) sit a few steps away from your cart. You have faithfully posted pics of your meals for the last few days. Now, a dilemma confronts you. If you purchase these cookies, you cannot sneak and eat them in the car on the way home like you usually would. You would be required to be honest, take a quick pic, and confess your sin. Should you show everyone how weak you are? Or, should you forgo the picture taking and sharing? After all, no one would know, and it is no one's business what you eat. Right? Well, of course. We reside in a free country, and chocolate chip cookies are not a punishable crime. You can hear the back and forth in your mind. In that instant, you experience the familiar feelings of hiding, shame, and not fulfilling your promise to yourself.

Is it worth it?

No. Cookies lose.

Now, we are getting somewhere.

Make the clock your best friend

We are going to turn TIME into your most powerful tool. Your watch will help you gain control over the minute-by-minute games of your mind. It gives us something to look forward to and helps us confront the automatic, non-stop, mindless eating we have become accustomed to in our prosperous first-world countries. If you are in the habit of eating breakfast, snack, lunch, snack, dinner, late-night snack, then you are probably reading this book because you are addicted to food.

We will use the clock to tell us when to eat, and the clock we are using will not say: eat at 7a, 10a, 12p, 3p, 6p, 9p, only to fall asleep and start the process over again tomorrow. We will use the clock to train ourselves to ultimately cram our eating into a 3-hour window while we are in "lose weight" beast mode. Intermittent fasting will not be a permanent state, but we will reset our new feeding clock to always return to it quickly and without much daily life disruption. We will break the clock that tells us to focus on what to eat daily.

Turning your struggle into a healthy hobby

You are still failing even though you know everything you need to know intellectually about the topic of how to "lose weight." You continue to falter in this area of your life, even if you are wildly successful at other things like work, hobbies, video games, celebrity gossip, google research, church, listening to music, fashion, hair, nails.

Eating is the most basic human activity. We come into this world, and one of the first things that we do (after crying, screaming, and wiggling around) is to find mom's breast for that first feed. Many early childhood memories link to food in the form of birthday cakes, Valentine's Day chocolate, Halloween candy, Thanksgiving turkey, Christmas cookies, school lunches, and snacks in the car's back seat.

Our world could be falling apart around us, and most of us would still be looking for what to put in our mouths and stomachs next.

For many of us, food means habits, routines, and emotions. Feelings about food confront us frequently throughout the day. Dealing with food may feel like a consuming (pun intended) state of moving through time and space.

Whatever conditions brought you to this book, I am confident that you can think through your life and pinpoint emotions and incidents that have shaped your self-image and body concept. You want to make improvements, and you will. We will. Together. I promise. Step one is understanding that these principles will take you through the rest of your life. The endpoint is when you leave this earth, and that is okay.

Generating a list of the best foods to eat today does not address the continuous mental struggle you are experiencing at this moment and will feel tomorrow. The food list does not always serve you because it leaves you placing your failure back in your lap when you stray from the list.

It is a lack of motivation, lack of discipline, lack, lack, lack that is causing you to stay stuck. All these thoughts torture and discourage you. Your mind is actively involved in sabotaging your plans. Curiously enough, none of these thoughts change you or keep you away from the brownies and cheesy nachos.

If you view this obsession as a problem today, you may as well admit that you will have this problem for the rest of your life. Instead of calling this problem a problem, we will rename it and call it a "healthy daily lifelong journey." Now we have a hobby and never-ending rabbit hole to explore and pursue. Does that not feel so much more exciting and interesting? It will if you stay with me.

A word on Covid-19

Social distancing. Quarantine. Empty grocery shelves. Curbside pickup. New normal.

Scared to go to the gym. Quarantine fifteen. Comfort food. Sitting in the car. Breathing and re-breathing your air, masked. Also, the new normal.

Public citizens everywhere are feeling the effect of Covid-19 on behavior, mood, and daily activities. Scientific and medical communities have done an excellent job conveying information that links Covid complications to the presence of comorbidities such as obesity, type 2 diabetes, and heart disease.

Although I am just a regular person trying to be healthy, I can see from the posts shared in my group how deeply concerned we "regular" folks are about boosting our immune systems and dropping extra, unwanted pounds. It is not easy to start or maintain a fitness routine from home during lockdowns. The struggle to eat healthy meals at home is real. Never have we seen a time in history when solving these weight-related health problems is so critical.

HOW to gain control of your body through the power of Time and Timing

Here is where we will spend most of our time. This book is about day-to-day, hour-to-hour, minute-to-minute strategies that will help you unpack your obsession with food and constant desire to eat. That is what has gotten you to this point, whether you have 20 pounds to lose or 80 pounds. We will confront the behavior of food obsession, weight gain, and loss in such a way that your mind and resulting actions become a tool to assist you rather than a weapon against your progress.

We will go deep into actions, strategies, and suggestions that will get and keep you motivated to move your body and ENJOY your workout routine. Gone are the excuses for procrastinating and pretending you do not know what to do to keep from being "bored" with exercise.

The secret power of intermittent fasting

When I strapped in and embarked on the challenge of posting and taking pictures of all my food in October 2016, I had no idea that it would lead me to intermittent fasting. All I wanted was a mechanism to be more accountable about what I was eating and find a way to control my secret and, at times, indulgent practices.

At that time, I had not committed to any particular WOE. The notion of showing my plates was enough to select "healthy" options instinctually. Due to my pride, I would not want to admit to taking a pic of fast-food garbage or a shareable bag of M&Ms that mysteriously is never shared. A lifetime of "dieting" knowledge kicked in. Veggies, proteins, small portions, small plates were the go-to starting points for what I could reasonably and proudly post.

I noticed several trends, all about tried-and-true dieting advice. Let's examine the adage, "drink water." How many magazine articles have we read telling us the key to losing weight is "drinking water"? Plenty, because this advice is standard and sounds reasonable enough.

However, drinking water is only part of a complex system of new habits you will have to build. Drinking water is not stand-alone advice. The only way you would know that this alone will not move the needle is if you try it. I suggest you follow the "drink water" advice for a period of, let's say, 30 days. The scale may not move, but drinking water is a foundational first floor in the intermittent fasting building.

Focusing on water is excellent advice if you, for example, have a soda pop addiction that is adding unnecessary calories. If that is the case, then yes, drink water instead of high-calorie carbonated beverages. Do not consume your calories. Calories are too precious to waste on liquids. Use water specifically as a substitution and habit-breaking tool. You can start to see how this kind of shift in thinking will bring you to a new understanding of conventional advice. It will also prevent you from being frustrated about why you are doing something like "drinking water" and not "losing weight."

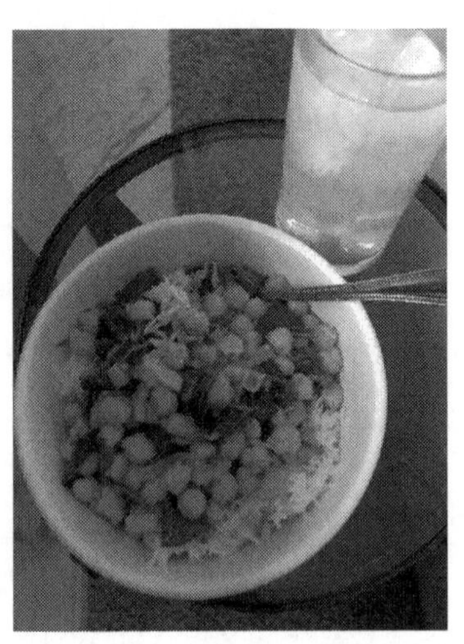

Drinking water is only one layer of the dieting onion. We will peel back layers you did not even know existed. I can help you do this because I have looked at every angle of this problem and may even discover more before I finish writing this book and long after.

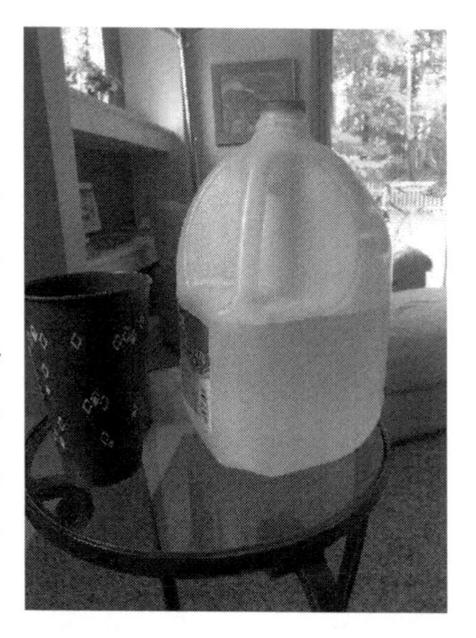

Over time, I gradually tried other WOEs. Sometimes I felt like not eating meat. Sometimes I felt like not eating carbs. Sometimes I felt like restaurant food and weekend cheats were a particular culprit. The list of habits to tackle seemed endless.

With each door I opened, more information came to the surface, and I realized that eating itself was a huge problem, as strange as that may sound.

Thoughts of specific foods cause you to think it is possible to create a magical list of items that will turn you into an underwear model if eaten in the proper combination. Guess what? This supernatural food list does not exist. Instead, the answer lies within your personalized system of habit changes that will support your daily strategies and turn your struggle into a fun and healthy obsession.

The more pics and posts I made, the more determined I was to find the silver bullet. I was becoming very aware of problem areas in my diet. I also had a front-row seat to the confessions of friends in the group. We all seemed to have similar struggles: sugary snacks, sketchy beverages, late-night eating, indulgent celebrations were among the common themes.

One miraculous day, I was chatting on the phone with a friend from my accountability group. He suggested that I investigate a medical doctor who teaches about intermittent fasting. My friend cautioned me that this particular medical doctor has somewhat of a dry and scientific presentation. Trusting my friend as a source, I looked this doctor up and dove into his content. Hours later, I was still listening.

The answer was simple: stop eating. Group members could solve all their problems by putting the fork down and removing all-day consumption tendency.

Enter intermittent fasting.

I advise you to research the science behind why intermittent fasting is so effective. This book's purpose is not to write a term paper from Google sources intended to convince you that "not eating" will cause you to lose weight. After all, is that not an obvious idea and one that does not need to be "proven"? Yes. It is simple. So simple that we have

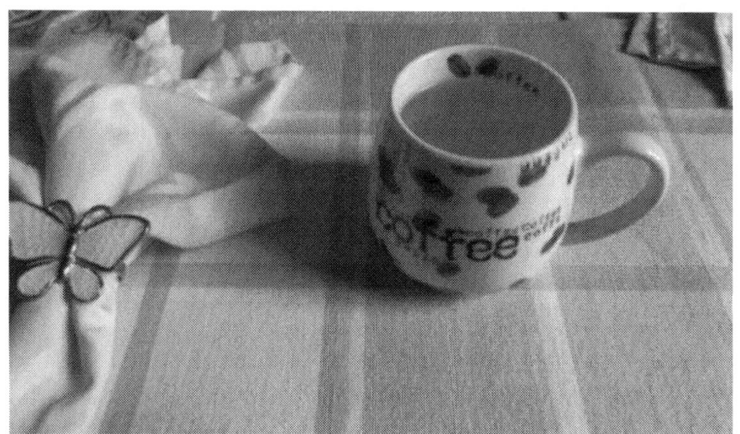

complicated it beyond what is necessary. If you desire the scientific evidence to justify intermittent fasting, please, by all means, go for it. Click over to the internet and type "intermittent fasting" into the search bar.

Did you find what you were seeking? Great.

For me, I only needed a few key new pieces of information. I learned that eating ANYTHING causes insulin levels to rise. Insulin is the culprit behind triggering the body to store fat. As long as insulin levels are up, you will continue to hold stored fat. Your body uses energy all day long. The trick is to get your system to use stored fat as its energy source. Body fat is your fuel. How do you get your body to burn itself? By not eating.

It took some time to digest the meaning behind this fully. All these years, I thought that my body was burning what I just ate. If I ate six times a day, and each item was low-calorie, indeed, I should be at a calorie deficit and would lose weight. Right? Well, no, because insulin levels are at a constant high throughout the day, and fat stores are constantly inaccessible.

The key was not in WHAT I was eating. It was the TIME I needed to spend NOT eating. While not eating, my body could enter the fat burn zone. Each hour in the fasted state was time spent "losing weight." I would turn off the fat-burning switch the minute I ate, even if I ate something low-calorie like an apple. The key is to keep the fat-burning button on as long as possible for as many days as possible until you burn all stored fat and become a lean, mean bikini machine.

Remove the notion that you should eat and burn off what you just ate, especially if you have stored fat on your body. Replace this notion with the concept of burning the fat cells that are already sitting happily under your skin.

Only by implementing this eating and not eating cycle could I see the results that would convince me of this particular strategy's power. The longer I delayed feeding, the more time my body would have to attack and use fat stores for energy.

Before learning of the role insulin plays in fat storage, I thought calorie counting, eating smaller meals, and eliminating entire food groups was the answer. Meanwhile, this was not working for me, and I could not figure out why. Perhaps deprivation only caused my mind to fixate on that eliminated food group. Maybe calorie counting was too much of an inexact and futile exercise. In actuality, eating throughout the day, even if the meals were "normal," never allowed my body time to access the fat stores that made me look more fluffy than lean.

Intermittent fasting removed all guesswork from my daily eating. Disregarding food entirely for a specified time naturally encouraged me to control myself during the feeding window. Another beautiful element of the intermittent fasting plan is cost: free.

The role of "calories" and what to eat in your feeding window

Another critical piece of information I learned was that sugar and processed carbs raise insulin levels higher than fat and protein. Good fats and protein, like avocado, nuts, and lean meats, cause feelings of fullness. The 100 calories good fat-rich avocado digests differently than a 100-calorie carb-rich hamburger bun. The burger bun raises your insulin level and knocks you out of fat-burning ketosis, causing you to store fat; the avocado helps you stay in ketosis. For the non-diet nerds reading this book, ketosis is a metabolic state of stored fat as energy.

Although I never expressly or strictly followed a ketogenic diet, I understand why keto and paleo are successful. As long as your body is in ketosis, you are fat burning. As an experiment, purchase keto strips from your local drug store to investigate how eliminating sugar from your diet affects your ketone levels. Keto works not because of calorie counting but because energy no longer comes from sugar-rich processed carbs.

Counting calories has become the gold standard activity in dieting. If you simply cannot turn your brain off from automatic calorie counting, simply change the focus. Eat the 100-calorie avocado instead of the 100-calorie processed snack food pack. The avocado will leave you feeling more satisfied. It is also harder to binge on avocados.

View calories in an entirely different way: to compare quality between foods. We have all heard that "less is more" when it comes to calories. We have not spent as much time on the notion that you can take in the same number of calories with higher quality foods and lose weight more efficiently than with the same number of low-quality foods.

When deciding what to eat during your window, keep the idea of not eating processed foods at the top of your priority list. Try also to eat whole raw foods, green veggies, and small amounts of fruits. Plant- or lean meat-proteins are ideal. You have developed your food preferences over your lifetime, and intermittent fasting allows you to honor what you like and enjoy as long as you spend more time during your day NOT eating than eating when in weight loss mode.

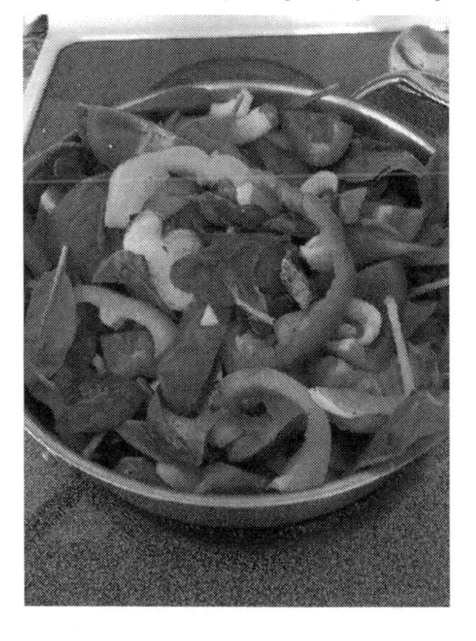

When I shared my food history, I mentioned a 5-year stint during my teen years when I became a semi-vegetarian. I ate fish and chicken, but no red meat. It is in my nature to prefer a plant-based or lean protein diet. The beauty of intermittent fasting is its adaptability.

Remember, this book is not about creating a stifling food list that will make you feel trapped and rebellious. This book is about changing your mindset around time spent NOT eating so that you can burn fat. When all the fat you have stored on your body burns off and disappears, you can move into the direction of maintenance and merely be comfortably aware of how your intake's timing affects the numbers on the scale.

A word on "feeling hungry": while fasting, I want you to know that I paid close attention and noticed that I did not ever really experience feelings of hunger. I had an annoying longing for food, similar to the feelings of missing a friend or activity that I enjoyed. Stick another pin in that whole thought. We will explore more later.

Doing what you say

How many times have you said, "I want to lose weight," or "I want to eat better," or "I want to start working out." Zillions.

Now pause and re-read those weak, vague statements. No wonder you have yet to achieve your goals.

The foundation of the *3 Hour Window Diet* is saying something particular about HOW you intend to proceed. There is nothing vague about a 3-hour intermittent fasting window. There is something to be said about simplicity.

Apply the concept of being specific about what you plan to do in everything related to your new lifestyle. Because you have chosen a team of accountable friends and family, you have plenty of sets of ears who will listen to you speak your specific plans. Over the past four years, I have written several volumes of statements related to what I am doing, have done, and plan to do. These statements are made on social media, in text messages, in conversations with fellow strugglers.

"I will take a step class at 6:15a on Monday and Wednesday of this week" provides far more precise instructions than "I will work out twice this week."

"I will eat a bowl of broccoli, as much as I want, well-seasoned, at 4p today" is better than "I'll grab something later." One statement captures your best intention. The other leaves you open to temptation and poor planning. Each time you fulfill your promise to yourself, you trust yourself more and more. Each statement builds on the previous. You figure out what is easy to do and what is more of a challenge.

Integrity within yourself means doing what you say you are going to do and keeping promises. Having a definitive plan and mindset is needed to get through the hours when you are not sleeping and not eating. Some days will be a struggle, some days a breeze. As long as you have more A+ days than F days, you will see improvements and progress.

The power of people and accountability, why AI and apps will not make you skinny

A fellow weight loss struggler friend said something that I found strange. She said, "accountability does not work for me." Her declaration shocked me, and I spent several days pondering what seemed to be an outrageous claim and perhaps even a feeble excuse. I realized that some folks view accountability as a process in which you rely and depend on another person to help get you where you need to be. When or if that person falls off, ghosts, or does not follow through, you feel that "accountability does not work."

There is a flaw in that thinking. Accountability does not mean you rely on someone ELSE to make you do food and fitness consistently. Instead, you eat properly, engage in fitness frequently, and share your activities with others. The other people's power comes when you tell them what you will do, and you feel hard-pressed to do it. They are bystanders in the movie starring you. They are your audience. Cheering and encouragement are the gas in your tank, especially when you feel weak and powerless during the worst cravings.

Since starting my private accountability group, *80/20 Journal*, I have prioritized staying abreast of weight loss trends. If you are reading or listening to this book, you may be aware that the trends are to "automate" and "scale" the process by employing a technology-based solution, often with a price tag. While these new tools boast some testimonial success, most of us would be far more successful with a real person involved in our accountability and not an automated digital assistant. This "sponsor" model has worked well for Alcoholics Anonymous, and we can employ it.

Is it only one person you need? No! You need an army of real people, some people you know, some you may not know. When you become consciously aware of the nuts and bolts of this problem and how it impacts your life, you will discover that you may need help more often than you ever realized.

When selecting your tribe of accountability buddies, I recommend choosing various people at different stages on the road to solving this problem. I have several circles. Women provide other feedback than men. Someone faithful to exercise will give more motivation than someone who has not seen the inside of a gym in years. A person who has lost over 50 pounds will provide a perspective that someone who cannot get past 5 pounds has never experienced. You can be in communication with all these people. Sometimes you will be the encourager; sometimes, you will encourage the other person. Both roles are significant. Give and take.

You should also evaluate your level of competitive energy. If you are competitive, it might help you to partner up with someone who is neck and neck with you in the race. Iron sharpens iron. Be wary of the energy you exchange with people who are not serious about making changes or reaching goals. Stay away from individuals who are always struggling, cannot keep a commitment, or give up easily. Do not allow anyone to derail you from your resolution to keep going.

The human mind's nuances are such that an automated response plan cannot give you everything you need. AI and apps can be 20% of your complete strategy. Instead, real people with real voices and real faces interacting with you in real-time will help you through the more impactful 80%.

Journaling: creating a separate and dedicated space

In our digital world, we are pushing more and more personal data into the cloud. Let's step away from the 0000s and 1111s and back in time to the analog space. Pick your head up from the screen for one moment.

Grab a pen and a piece of paper.

Write, do not type, a statement that you wish to be true about yourself related to your weight loss end-game.

Here is my statement: "Glenda, you are your goal weight of 140lbs. You are never, I repeat, never, going to drift past 145. It's okay. 5-pound swing weight is completely adequate for you to live life yet still look and feel amazing on your 5'3 ½" frame. It is time to STAY where you have always wanted to be."

Writing is an incredibly underutilized weight loss goal-setting tool.

When I went through my trunk looking for old pictures, I discovered journal entries from my 20s in which there were notes and entries about what I had eaten for the day and my workouts. Keeping this issue in front of my mind fostered a desire to share my passion with others by teaching fitness.

Reminder: you cannot help people lose weight if you have never done it yourself. If you have not developed a unique set of tools that have worked long term, you cannot give someone a set of meal plans and wish them good luck on their merry way.

Most people's weight loss failure is that they do not take it seriously enough or implement enough strategies to move outside the fantasy realm. Making detailed charts will force you out of weight loss dreamland and into success and achievement.

Now that you have written a goal statement for what you want, let's turn to the reality of what IS.

If you are reading or listening to this book, I guarantee you do not remember 80% of what you ate last week. We are going to change that. Step 1 to changing your situation is acknowledging the problem. Take your ostrich head out of the sand. Confront what you eat and its damage on the scale and in the mirror today.

Under your goals, write what you ate today, and continue this log for the next seven days. Write down every morsel of every item that passes your lips. The purpose of this exercise is to remove and eliminate the mindless eating you have been doing that has gotten you to the point of needing to read *3 Hour Window Diet*. Add pictures to your camera roll to pack a punch to this experiment. You are not required to share your journal and pics for the first seven days. We will keep it between us for now.

Over these next seven days, open your eyes to your problem areas.

Let's get started.

weight	Day 1 of 30	steps	gym	food	fasting hours
	Day 2				
	Day 3				
	Day 4				
	Day 5				
	Day 6				
	Day 7				

Scheduling and routine

When I started the online accountability group, the first promise I made to myself was not that I would "lose weight." Instead, I decided to post a "good morning" message at 6:00a Eastern Standard Time, welcoming the group participants to the new day and sharing a positive affirmation.

The good-morning post idea was my first step in using the clock as a primary tool. I set my cell phone alarm for 5:55a, allowing 5 minutes to ponder my reflection for the group. I had to force my brain into a positive and encouraging thought space before my feet hit the floor to make my bed. I also adopted a habit of documenting my progress by counting the days, weeks, and months we were active in this fight.

"Good morning, team 80/20! Welcome to month 2, week 6, day 4. Be your best by doing your best today."

Four years later, I still have a daily habit of posting something to the group that chronicles my healthy lifestyle habits.

But it all started with that 6:00a clockwork "good morning" and positive affirmation. Members could set their alarms to this notification, and it set me on the right track for the day.

Often, throughout the day, I would remind myself of what I had posted to the group in the early morning. These mental reminders helped build the muscle of remaining upbeat and positive while trying to stay on the path to do something that many of us find difficult.

As a first step, try this 6:00a good morning exercise for 30 days and see how it frames your day and gets you on your new hyper-vigilant clock. Send that good morning text to your sister in another state, your best friend from college, your son in the next room. It does not matter who receives the message. Make a list of 10 people you want to reconnect with, and send each one a new message over the next ten days. Repeat that sequence until 30 days is complete. It may seem silly; it may seem cheesy. That is fine if it looks that way or feels that way. Do it anyway if you want to harness your thinking and thoughts. Transform your mind before you lose the first pound. A specific plan to focus on yourself daily is a foundational building block.

Planning

The downfall of every dieter is the failure to plan. When you do not have a plan in place, you are under the grip of your constant whims of temptation and appetite. You may not even be hungry, but you can dream up thoughts of something you absolutely must eat right now. Admit it.

Step one of planning is getting more specific than you have ever gotten in your life. Saying "I want to lose weight" is not a plan. "Losing weight" is just words, if not followed up by a million actions. The specific work to "lose weight" is work that you must do, not work that someone else has done or should do for you. All the work is personal. The moment you try to push the work into another person's lap, you are walking down the wrong path.

Let's take meal planning as an example. When you download a meal plan, 9 out of 10 times, you may follow it the first day, then let the meal plan stay on your hard drive or phone and never open it again. Why would you? You did not create it specifically for you based on your preferences. All you did was download it.

Try something different. Review several plans to gather information to create your personalized meal plan that you will follow for seven days and seven days only. Write the customized meal plan down in your journal. The vital task and the goal task are to do what you said you would do for seven days straight.

You "hold yourself accountable" to this plan by eliciting the support of a few friends or family members. Tell them what you plan to do for the next seven days. Tell them that you may need to contact them when you consider deviating from the plan and what you will want from them in those moments. Tell them you will need them to talk you off the ledge and give you tough love. Tell them they have permission to check in with you later to see if you fulfilled your promise.

It is this level of detailed planning that will help you "lose weight." Part of what we are building is a framework of continuous actions to keep you engaged.

Not only will you build actions for what you can or want to eat during your feeding window, but you can get very creative with these activities to take your mind off food.

You will approach working out with the same high level of precision and detail depending on your current activity level. As I mentioned, I am a former fitness instructor and have always enjoyed working out. First, assess what your tolerance is for exercise. Are you primarily inactive? Or do you have a minimum level of commitment that you would like to increase and expand? If you are reading this book, you likely either struggle with starting a workout plan or sticking to one.

Again, using the anchor of the calendar and clock, you will make your 30-day workout plan. Whatever your current level is, commit to increasing your workouts for specific times and days. Change your plan every month, always keeping it fresh and improving. Over the four years of reporting activity, my list of "go-to" options for exercise is exhaustive. There is no opportunity to make excuses. All you can do is increase and improve.

In 2019, I had a one-week vacation from work. I set a personal fitness goal for my staycation: walk 100,000 steps in one week. Because I had never done anything like this, it seemed like a tall order and big commitment. I set out to walk 20k steps 5 of 7 days. For my height, average speed, and stride length, walking 20k steps takes about 2 hours. It was a challenge to find a course that would give me enough steps.

Once I got comfortable with a particular route, I immediately changed it to provide myself with different scenery and stay engaged in the commitment. I told my group what I planned and posted screenshots of my steps each day.

Members of the group were incredulous. Once someone shows you an idea, it inspires you to try it also. Since that step challenge, several group members have picked up the same activity, and many regularly report similar outrageous step counts, mileage, and intense workouts. The simple act of beginning to record and observe your data can motivate you and others to do more.

The 100k step challenge opened the door to a habit that I continued into 2020. Now, I regularly walk 6 miles at one shot.

Once you start, you cannot stop.

Living your life during non-feeding hours is the key to strengthening your overall loss plan.

And you must start somewhere.

Penalties and rewards

One of the reasons you are having difficulty sticking to a plan is that you have not given yourself concrete incentives or penalties that work. Your motivations probably sound something like: "I would like to look great in a bathing suit." Or, "I cannot wait to buy a whole new wardrobe when I drop a few sizes."

Those daydreamy vision statements sound sufficient enough. Yet, here we are, months and years later, still in the same place.

Why is that? Well, your daydreamy statements are too far into the future. Looking great in a bathing suit is a wishful thought in November when it is getting cold outside. Buying a whole new wardrobe is not a big deal when you have clothes to wear today; even if you do not feel you look your best, you do not walk around naked.

This book is about flipping conventional practices upside down. Instead of planning to celebrate success far into the future where you cannot see it, receive your reward today. Post a picture of a beautiful, healthy meal and enjoy the feedback from friends and family who compliment your plating skills or encourage you to continue working on your healthy diet goals. The immediate reward is in the positive feedback and engagement your support squad provides every step of the way. Enjoy the interaction when someone asks you a question about what you are eating, how your meal tastes, or what you did to prepare it. Give yourself an impromptu platform to speak the words of commitment to yourself and others.

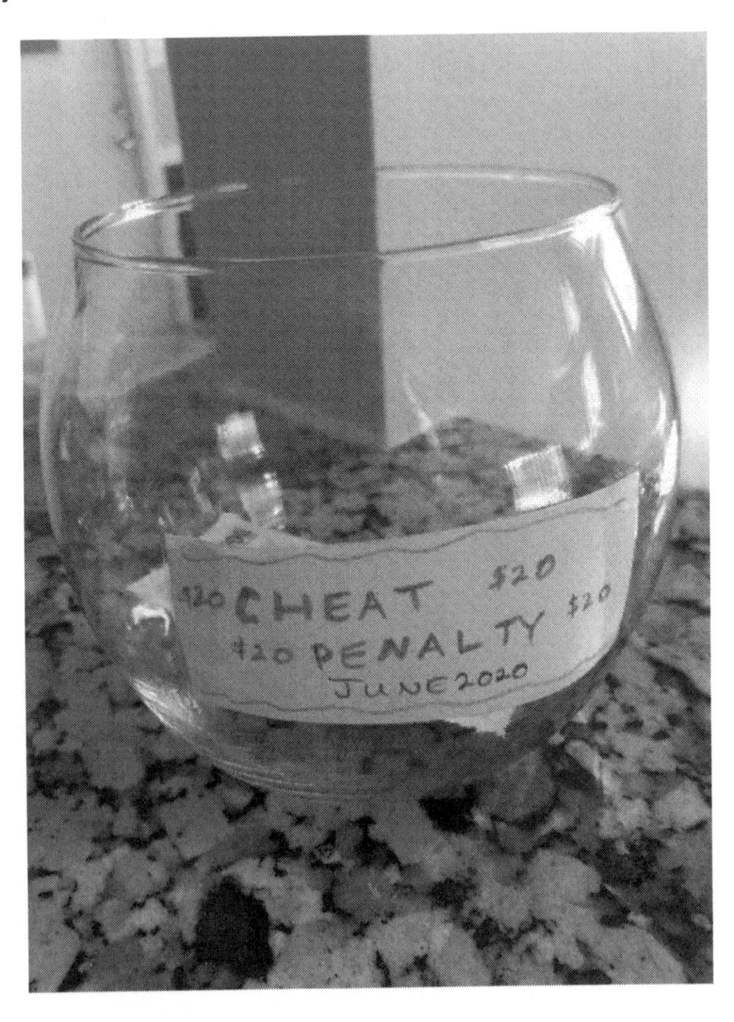

Your persona becomes synonymous with someone who makes their health a priority. How can you fail when you are developing the person you want to become today, rather than waiting for a bathing suit reveal (you can still do that, by the way)?

One month, I decided I needed some additional support to reach my goals. Online friends were helping immensely, but I needed some eyes on me in real life. Enter, my sons. I appointed them food police, and they were more than happy to oblige, especially my younger son Joseph. I made a penalty jar and put it on the counter. At that time, my 30-day commitment to myself was that I could go without cheating 100%. I had never made such a specific plan to defeat the cheat monster. If I had even a single cheat food, I had to put $20 in the penalty jar and split the money between my sons at the end of the month. It worked! That month, I only cheated once. Losing $20 was not worth it, but I was happy it was not $60 or $200.

True story: the real penalty of not following through on your plan is that you stay stuck, gain weight, feel bad. That is the constant penalty that you are enduring for years on end. Yet, somehow, that penalty is not enough to correct your behavior. Therefore, try a different incentive and watch it work.

If you are not motivated by putting money into a jar, try something else. What is your most hated household chore? Not a fan of taking out the trash in your home? Do you prefer to assign that task to a child or spouse? Penalty: YOU take out the garbage if you cheat. Write a chart and put it on the refrigerator so that everyone in the house knows that brownie will cost you. Small fun penalties and rewards will make your new lifestyle entertaining, bearable, and continuously motivating.

Changing it up

If you have tried to lose weight, you know that this monkey will possibly be on your back for the rest of your life. And guess what? That is okay! You are learning how to enjoy this process. A key component is not getting "bored." Let's be honest. Nothing is boring about losing weight if you are losing it. Boring is: starting a plan, failing on the first day, restarting tomorrow, falling flat on your face two days after that, restarting on day 4, giving up on day 6, then stepping on the scale, and being distraught that the numbers are going in the wrong direction. Super boring.

Why does this happen? Because your plan is nebulous, and it does not have enough "components."

Think about every so-called diet you have ever attempted. You probably remember some foods you were allowed to eat and more that were off-limits. Perhaps you remember a magic number of calories ideal for daily consumption. After you tried this "diet" or, ah-hem, "way of eating," you tapped out. You had reached the end of the road, and you had not even made it through the first week.

Does this sound familiar? Even if you were able to stick to your plan for ten days or two weeks, at some point, you needed something else.

3 Hour Window Diet is different because there is no limit to what foods you can try within your 3-hour window based on your preferences. We are staying wedded to *the clock,* as it provides a stable foundation for your structured eating plan, not the foods inside your window.

Since you already know what to eat and what not to eat, what you like and what you do not like, there is no need to focus on that list or rely on anyone else to provide you with a plan that will not suit your needs. Instead, focus on the clock.

What time are you eating today, and when will you start preparing? What do you need to do to stay on course before that hour strikes? What will you do after the window is closed before you go to bed? The clock, the clock, the clock. Give yourself enough flexibility within reason inside of your window. Outside of your window, focus your battleplan on staying strong doing activities that will keep you away from breaking away from your plan.

Knowing your destination helps you create a roadmap to get there. There is no need to be concerned that you will give up the first week because your mission is to work your way up to this point, come back to it when necessary. You are strength training and flexing your fasting muscle. Try something within your window for the first week. Depending on your results, you can always tweak or make changes, even with the 3 hours you pick. I often start my 3-hour window at 4p. On days that I felt like I needed a change, I simply adjusted the start time of my window, and boom, I feel different yet still engaged in the process.

Pictures, pictures and more pictures

If you find that you are always turning sideways to take pictures, it's time.

If you only take selfies, you need to get yourself together.

If you keep recycling and reposting old pictures from when you were thinner, it is time to update your look by fixing what you secretly want to improve.

If you are relying on angles to correct the truth, you have come to the right spot.

Use your camera to speak the truth and shame the devil.

Commit to taking several photos that will help you track your progress: before pics, scale pics, and side-by-side comparison pics. Use these pics, not for vanity, but as a tool to use when you feel like turning back from your path.

For example, when you wake up in the morning before you jump out of bed, pick up your phone (you do this anyway), and scroll through your scale pics from the previous month. If you feel a lack of motivation to get up and make that morning workout happen, this simple action can be the much-needed nudge.

Many of your bad habits stem from the repetitive, unhelpful foods you frequently eat. Let's say Mickey Ds is your weakness. You have been taking pics of all your food for seven days, and the habit has stuck.

Now you are on week 4 of taking pics of your food. You look through your camera roll and see 4 Mickey Ds pics in 4 weeks. Time to issue yourself a challenge. No fast food for the next 30 days. If you had not taken pics and reviewed them, your mind would not have that concrete evidence staring at you from your screen.

The truth will set you free! You need to have a strategy to implement and review the truthful evidence of the eating patterns that held you back. You are beginning to see why a *3 Hour Window Diet* is so much more than a list of recommended plant-based proteins and ways to spice up kale and quinoa.

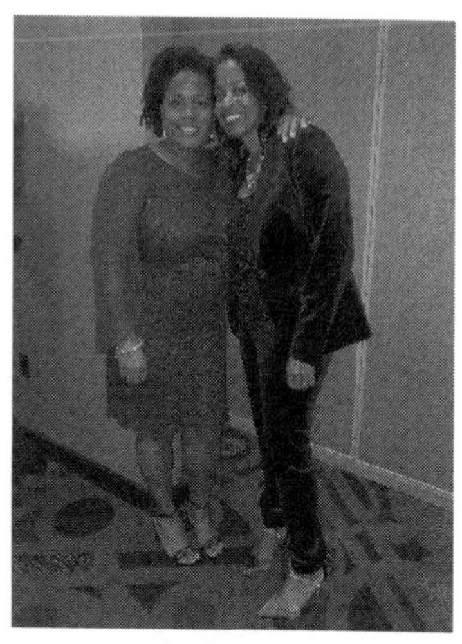

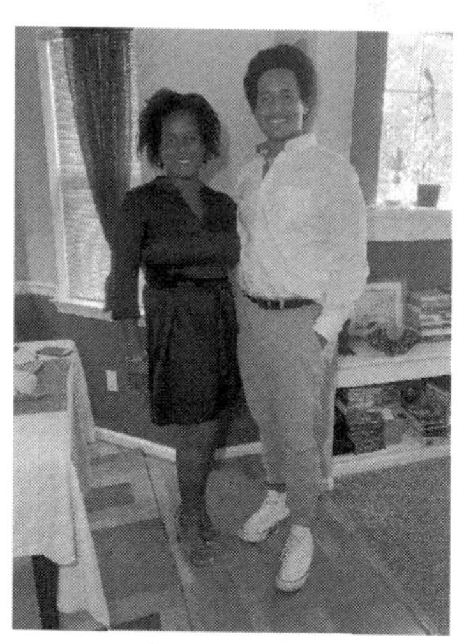

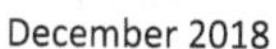

December 2018

September 2020

Feel the feelings

On October 28, 2020, I made the following post in my private group:

"Good morning, team 80/20! I just experienced a strange situation. Those who have been participating in or observing our group know that I'm an early riser, the preferred time of day to workout/walk is early morning. I firmly believe that getting it out of the way in the AM is the best antidote to the procrastination urge that kicks in the PM.

This morning, rather than setting out for the track or trail early, I decided to sit in my living room in front of the morning news, FB, and online information. I was curious about the coverage of Philadelphia's situation because my son John is an online student at Temple University.

During this un-normal session of depressing news consumption, I became overwhelmed with a craving for garbage breakfast. Images of Chik-fil-A and Dunkin hit me. Ugh! Like the cravings were so intense, I had to pause and think about where this was coming from seriously??

In my self-analysis, I diagnosed that media consumption left me feeling bummed. What would be the fix? Eating something "yummy." Emotional eating. Horrible.

What did I do? Put on my workout clothes and headed to the track for fresh air and movement therapy. Moral of the story: watch your triggers and avoid them. We all agree that 2020 has been a hot mess. Stick to (or start) habits that feed your body and soul rather than take away from your positive mental.

Make it a great day."

Here is your mission for today and the next few days. The next time you get hit by a powerful desire to eat something unhealthy, stop and take note of what you are doing and feeling at that very moment. Note a brief narrative of your dilemma in your journal. Do something physical to arrest the urge and change your thoughts. Ten jumping jacks, put your sneakers on, take a 5-minute walk outside, do ten squats. Try this exercise any time you feel a craving over the next week. Now you have a mechanism in place to remove rather than give in to the desire.

Resetting your feeding window

This plan is about more than food because you are weak in the face of food. Instead, you will use other tools that feel simpler and more neutral in providing the basis and harness around the new habits you are creating.

Let's examine how to use the clock and time as one of your new best friends. Recall, my first commitment to myself was the daily 6:00a posting to the group. You can develop, strengthen, and cultivate a relationship with the clock as a weapon in your new arsenal.

Right now, more than likely, you have no feeding clock. You are eating at random times during the day, at the mercy of every little thought, impulse, and craving.

Your commitment to the clock will be what time you plan to eat inside your first intermittent fasting window. Three hours is the goal, but it is not the starting line. Perhaps you may try starting with an 8-hour feeding window. Tell the clock your first meal will be 10a, and your last bite will be 6p. Watch the clock and honor it. You are forcing yourself to delay and cut off your feeding. At first, this practice will be a challenge. Over time, it will become natural and comfortable.

Select a feeding window that is unique to your schedule and typical food weaknesses. When I delay feeding until evening, it eliminates the muffin, bagel, sandwich carb-rich temptations of breakfast and go-to sandwiches for lunch. I am an early riser. Scheduling a morning workout in the fasted state bumps up the fat burn process. Later in the day, opening my feeding window after the morning workout and staying busy with errands is the grounded and staple routine. I do not mind deviations, but I always go back to the foundation. Establish your foundation, and build upward from there.

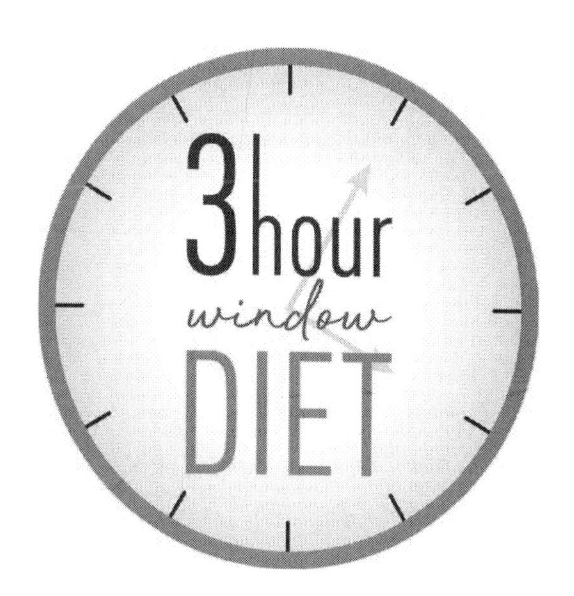

Not cheating

After recording your food consumption patterns, your habits will emerge. For me, I noticed that I could feel in control of my Monday through Friday regimen, but by the time Friday evening arrived, I felt like I deserved a break.

Enter: cheat weekends. Cheat weekends derailed my progress far too long. Had I started with intermittent fasting during the week, I might have been able to get away with some cheat weekends. Before I found intermittent fasting, I blindly followed the advice of eating three meals and two small snacks during the week. If I had been relatively "good" with my choices, I would feel I had a license to have happy hour drinks and wings, Saturday morning pancakes, Sunday family dinner followed by dessert. No wonder the scale was not moving, even though I was making a steady effort.

Those of us in the dieting community have heard of notations like 5:2, which means you do some form of fasting for five days straight, then take two days off. Let's examine the basis of this approach to weight management. We use the clock and calendar to grab hold of time and make it serve us, rather than feeling trapped by how much time has passed with no progress. Time is the variable we seek to control. However, if you cheat every five days, you are worse off than if you cheat once in 30 days.

Try this simple exercise. If you allowed yourself a total of 12 cheat meals in one year, which meals would you choose? Write it down! One month I penciled in my cheat for the last day of the month. By the time I reached that final day of the month, I was not even interested in eating that particular meal. I had a successful month; why ruin it? The action of simply writing down the cheat and telling myself I could have it on the last day of the month was enough to keep me focused on that month's finish line.

Challenges

We figured out early that once we got into the habit of taking pics and posting, we needed more structure on what we were posting and how our individual goals differed. Some wanted to focus on consuming enough water daily. Some had a loud sugary snack sweet tooth. Others felt confident in their food choices but struggled with the motivation to start and maintain an exercise schedule.

After about one month of journaling and recording meals and activities, you should have a good idea about creating a personal plan and challenging your weak areas one at a time. Using the calendar, set a goal for seven days, and consider yourself successful when completing that cycle. You will find that seven days is longer than it seems when you are attempting to kick an ingrained habit. You will gradually increase your challenge period to 14 days, 21 days, one month, and beyond.

Here are some of the challenges and teams we executed in our group with great success:

No Sugary Snacks

No Sketchy Beverages

Water Goals

Workout

No Fast Food

No Receipts (no eating out)

Plant-based Meals

30 DAY CHALLENGE

- No burger
- No chips
- No ice cream
- No fast food
- No chocolate
- No white bread
- No soda
- No cakes or donuts
- No cookies or candy

CHALLENGE SOMEONE

For days on end, rhythm of the calendar

Strategies are endless for how to stay motivated. Our family's kitchen calendar is a visual reminder of what I am focusing on for the month. How many days did I successfully stick to my 3-hour window? How many days did I hold off and break my intermittent fast at 4p? How many days did I hit our home garage gym? Record, record, record. Make it visible and plain to your household. There were moments when I felt weak and on the verge of caving. In those moments, simply walking over to the kitchen calendar and making a notation was enough to pull me back from slipping and falling. Try it. Everyone in your home will support your goals if you share them. No one can help you if you are quiet and daydreaming in your head.

Holidays and Seasonality

One of our group's faithful members posted this in response to a meme: "Train derailed Labor Day Weekend. My main goal in the final quarter of the year is to maintain any progress I've made that year. Between Labor Day Weekend, Halloween, my birth week, Scorpio season, Thanksgiving, Christmas, NYE, and shorter days/less sunlight, I consider it a win if I can keep the gain at less than 5lbs." I chuckled while reading this post.

This member is allowed to make these allowances because she also works out twice daily. If your activity level is not this high, you may want to reframe your approach to holidays so that you do not take an extended hiatus annually.

When you have completed an annual cycle, you will notice that food and activity preferences may shift with the seasons. In 2020, I found it was much easier to lose weight during the summer because of salad season and outdoor fitness. As chillier weather approaches, I will tighten my intermittent fasting practices to compensate for missing my 6-mile outdoor trail walks.

Annual goals

You are making small, detailed, specific changes every day that will support your long-term weight loss and weight maintenance goals.

One of our faithful group members shared a challenge early in 2020. Her gym would give a t-shirt to any member who successfully clocked in at the gym 150 times. Many of us made an annual commitment to work out whatever number of times we thought we could manage. I felt confident that I could commit to 5 workouts per week or 260 total workouts. I met that goal well in advance of December 31, 2020. By October, I hit 260 sessions and had to revise my annual goal number.

Week 1. Make a list of friends or loved ones with whom you will share your plans to embark on a healthy eating and fitness plan. Set the alarm and text one person on your list every morning at 6:00a to say good morning and something positive for you or that person. Example: "Good morning, friend. Make it a courageous and intentional day." Do this for 365 days. Do not skip a single day.

Week 2. Write down everything you eat and drink for seven days straight. Do not skip a single item that passes your lips.

3. Drink half your body weight in ounces daily for seven days straight.

4. Eliminate sugary snacks from your diet for seven days straight.

5. If you eat meat, have a plant-based dinner every evening for seven days straight.

6. Eat all your meals at home for seven days straight. Do not purchase any food on the road, not even a $1 cup of coffee from 7-11.

7. Make seven new meals (one per day, breakfast, lunch, or dinner) from recipes you have not previously tried.

8. Try seven mono-veggie meals for one week. For example, dinner is a large bowl of spinach (as much as you want). Other meals that day can be whatever you choose.

9. If you have never tried intermittent fasting, start with an 8-hour window. The first meal is at noon, and the last meal is 8 pm. Do this for seven days.

10. Prepare a 7-day supply of veggie soup. Eat this soup daily at 4p as your first meal of the day.

11. Eliminate white foods for seven days straight: no bread, flour, foods, pasta, potatoes, or rice.

12. Start your day's eating with one serving of fruit only for seven days. Do not eat your usual cereal, muffin, donut, or bagel breakfast.

13. Eliminate animal proteins from all meals for seven days straight. This suggestion is different than #5.

14. Purchase or make a 7-day supply of green juice. Substitute one meal of choice daily with your green juice.

15. Pick seven veggies that are not on your regular go-to list. Add each veggie to a meal daily for seven days.

16. If you regularly drink soda, coffee, caffeinated tea, alcohol, or energy drinks, eliminate them for seven days.

17. For seven days straight, do not eat anything after 6p

18. For seven days, eat a minimum of one meal daily seated at your kitchen or dining room table. Be mindful of meals you are eating standing up, in the car, at your desk, on the couch.

19. For a full calendar month, pick a food item or beverage that is a problem food for you and eliminate it. Examples: bread, sugary snacks, meat, alcohol. The purpose is to test and build your resolve around breaking habits.

20. For a full calendar month, eliminate fast food, pizza, convenience restaurants. If you regularly eat out at work, this will require planning and packing food from home in advance.

21. For seven days, break your intermittent fast at 2p and close your feeding window at 8p.

22. For seven days straight, consume only water as your beverage. This suggestion is different than #3.

23. For a full calendar month, record all food and beverages in your journal.

24. For seven days straight, take pictures of all food and beverages consumed. Do not skip any items and capture all portions.

25. For one calendar month, prepare at minimum two new meals at home using healthy recipes found online or in cookbooks.

26. For seven days, break your intermittent fast at 4p, close your feeding window at 7p.

27. Wake up every morning at 6 am and take a walk in your neighborhood. Do this for seven days straight.

28. Purchase a wearable apparatus for your workouts, such as a waist trainer, weighted vest, water backpack, heavy

hands, or ankle weights. Train with your wearable equipment three times a week for one calendar month.

29. Select an exercise of choice. If you are currently not exercising at all, set a goal of 2 workouts per week for 30 days. If you regularly exercise twice a week, increase that to 4 times per week for 30 days. If you regularly exercise 4 times per week, increase that to 6 times for 30 days. The idea is to increase your output and sustain that for 30 days.

30. Focus on one body part, for example, abs, upper body, lower body. Research spot exercises for that area of the body. Work that area 3 times per week for four weeks. Continue regular walking in addition to this spot training.

31. Purchase an inexpensive piece of workout equipment, such as an ab roller, resistance bands, stability ball, or jump rope. Research exercises for that piece of equipment. Use it four times weekly for one calendar month.

32. Determine and commit to the total number of workouts you can achieve in one calendar year. For example, if you think you can work out four times per week, set your annual number at 4x52=208.

33. Take a selfie every time you work out. Log 30 selfies. Journal how long it takes to complete this task. Challenge

yourself to complete it in the least amount of calendar days possible based on your fitness level.

34. Find a nearby high school track with a stadium and work out by walking up the stadium stairs. Log how many flights of stairs you complete. Increase by 10% each activity for 30 days. Record the number of floors you complete each time.

35. Add light hand weights (2-5lbs) to a walking workout. Complete four heavy-hands walks per week for one calendar month.

36. Locate an outdoor space to do a workout. Your activity can be walking, running, bodyweight exercises. The key is to locate an area outdoors, away from the home or gym. Train in that space four times weekly for one calendar month.

37. Organize a small group of friends or family members. Commit to reporting and sharing all workout activities for one calendar month. Keep the group intentionally tightknit so that no one can avoid or miss reporting.

38. Use a stand-alone fitness tracker, the one that comes standard with your phone or a downloadable app. Screenshot your daily activity for one calendar month. Transpose any data that is important to you to your hard copy journal. For example, I record the number of floors I

walk to track how many times I do a stair workout at the local high school track. Try to improve that data point.

39. Select a quick exercise such as push-ups, crunches, or squats. Pick a goal number of reps that would be safe but challenging for you to complete daily for one calendar month: for example, ten squats daily for a beginner.

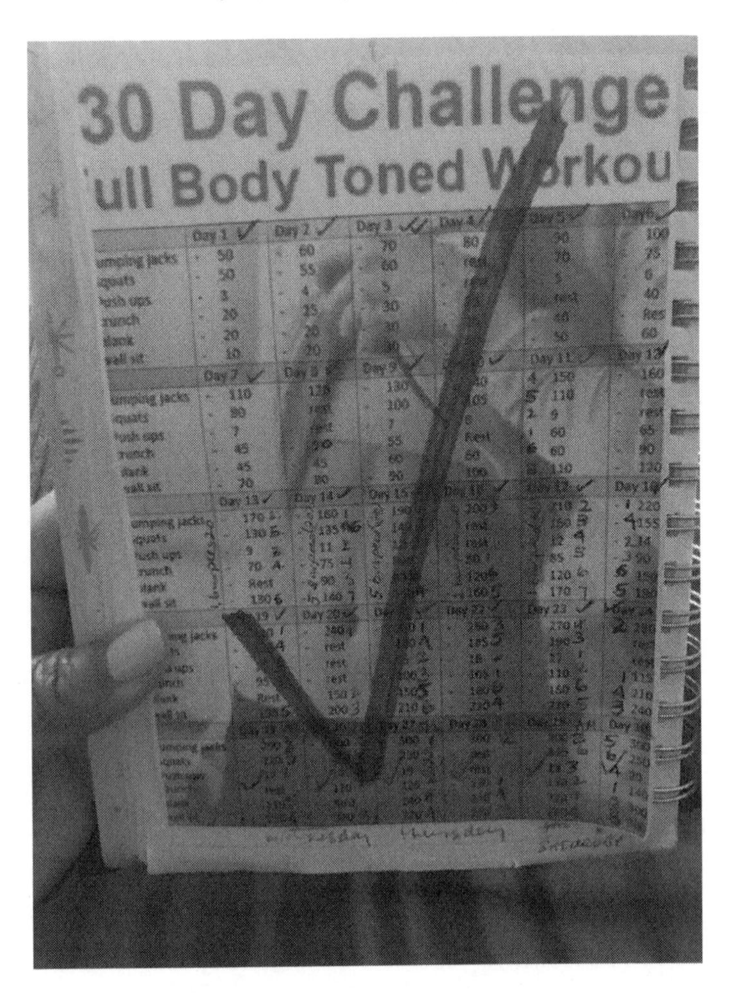

40. Pick a few friends or family members and do an in-person workout with that person at least twice a week for one calendar month.

41. Replace one meal with a workout three times per week for one calendar month.

42. Adopt the phrase "never-miss-a-Monday." When planning your workout schedule for the week, make sure you work out on Monday to get the week off to a good start.

43. Put a glass jar in a common area. Label the pot: "Workout Rewards." Put a dollar in the jar each time you work out. Watch the jar fill up. Make it rain!

44. Double your standard workout time three times in 7 days. If you regularly dedicate 30 minutes, increase your time to 60 minutes. If you usually log 60 minutes, go for 2 hours. Split the session if your schedule does not allow a continuous double block (1-hour workouts, twice in one day).

45. Take a picture from your workout of sneakered feet at the track or in the gym. Log 30 gym sneakers pics.

46. Follow an online or downloadable routine through an app. Do this three times over seven days. Workouts can be strength training, bodyweight resistance, or dance.

47. Try a 10-minute workout three times per day for four sessions for seven days.

48. Make a custom fitness "mixtape." Select fast-paced music and move in beat with your mix. Do not slow down.

49. Purchase a fitness or food-related audiobook. Listen to it while you work out. Complete the audiobook in as little time as possible, depending on your fitness level. For example, if the book's listening time is 8 hours, attempt to complete it in less than two weeks.

50. Purchase enough workout gear to take you through one full week of workouts without having to do laundry. Believe it or not, the need to do laundry can be a procrastination tool used by your mind to skip a workout.

51. Pick one day during the week and do a physical workout that is more functional, such as yard work, raking, gardening, house cleaning. Make sure you pay particular attention to your range of motion: reaching, squatting, bending, stretching.

52. Over seven days, walk 100,000 steps. When I did this challenge, I rested for two days and walked 20k steps daily for five days.

Presentation

When you put thought and beauty into designing a plate of colorful and nutritious items, you automatically become mindful of the nutrients entering your body. Have you ever studied the appearance of a salad filled with rich and vibrant cucumbers, red, yellow, and green peppers, purple onions, brown mushrooms, leafy green lettuce? It is truly magnificent.

Consider also how you serve your food. Pay attention to plating, silverware, placemats, tablecloths, drinkware. I change my table setting four times per year to complement the current seasons. Eating on real plates will feel very different than eating out of a bag or with plastic forks. Simple actions such as this will focus your inner attention on fully respecting your body's sustenance process.

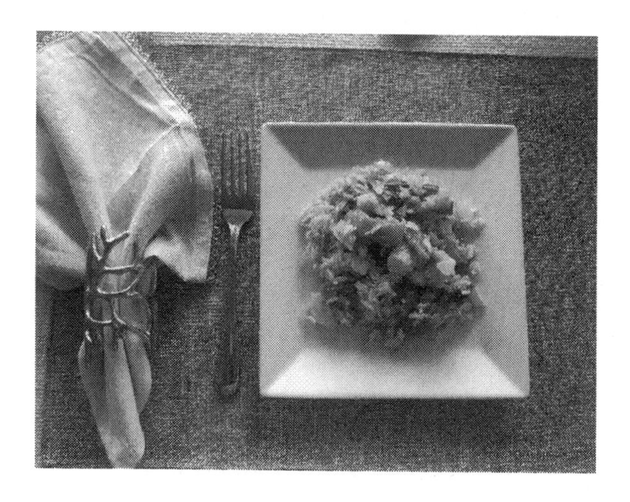

Fun and positivity

Here is an F word we rarely associate with "dieting": FUN. Once you form your group of accountability friends and family, make sure you include humor in your communications. Sharing memes, videos, emojis, and pictures will lighten the mood and help you look forward to trying new veggies or attempting additional reps in your strength training workout.

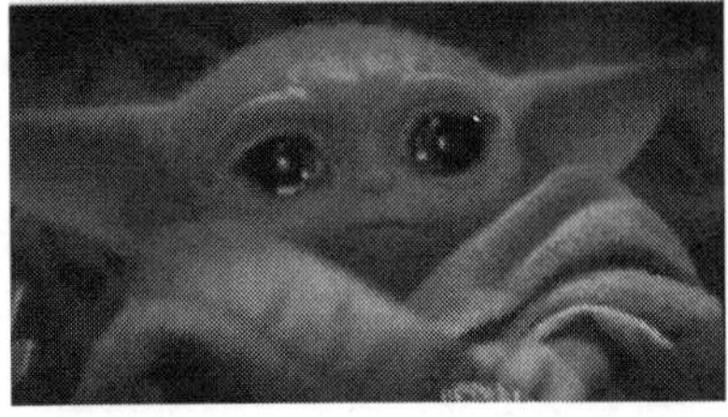

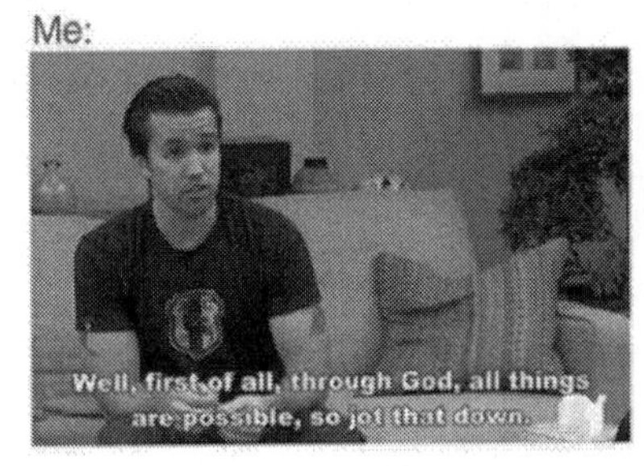

Simple affirmations will get you over a craving hump or temporary bout of workout laziness.

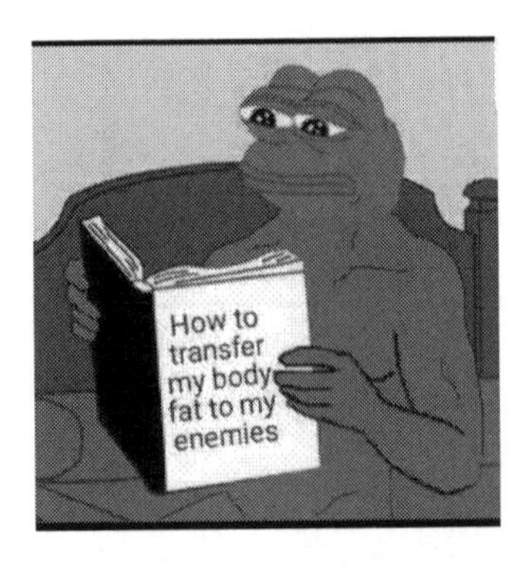

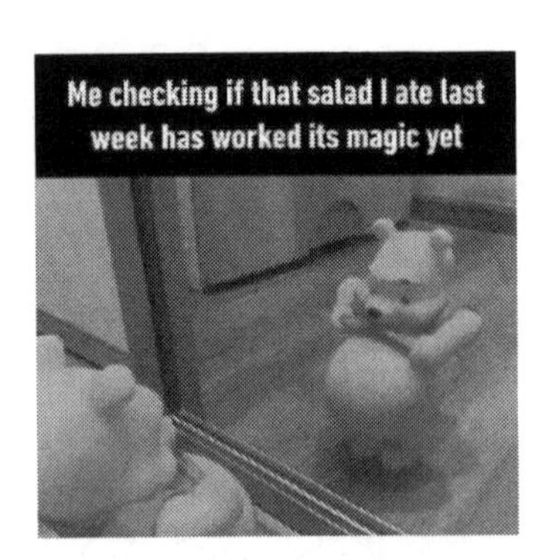

Videos, experts, gurus, podcasts

Now that you are getting accustomed to shorter feeding windows, you must develop a plan to stay mentally focused on continually consuming information to expand your knowledge of nutrition and fitness. There is no limit to what you can learn and what you do not know.

Remember the theme of this book. We are turning conventional practices upside down. The key to this part of the experiment is to use information as food that keeps you full while not eating. The purpose is NOT to find out something new that you can use to beat other people over the head or convince them of a particular practice.

Let me explain. We all know that friend who recently turned vegan. She or he has been vegan for about two weeks and keeps telling you why you must also become vegan. This person is annoying. Do not be like this person.

Instead, go to podcasts and videos and learn about the vegan lifestyle that works for those who choose it. Get lost in the podcasts. Yet another hour has passed that you did not spend in the kitchen shoveling unnecessary carbs before you know it.

What you learned on the podcast is secondary to filling the clock with non-food activities. Whether or not you become a vegan is tertiary to time spent in the fasting zone.

You have a phone next to you or have your laptop or digital reading device in front of you. You can turn these tools into sources of inspiration and information to keep you on point during your non-eating periods. If you do not, you will find your mind wandering (into food fantasy land), and that is what we are seeking to change.

Scale: friend or foe

I will start by proclaiming my position on the scale: I love you, I hate you, I need you, I despise you. While some follow the school of thought that states you should not weigh yourself, I reject that notion almost as much as I refuse strict calorie counting. Why? Because my progress is night and day when I check the numbers vs. when I do not. Therefore, I must make the scale my friend so that she can help me.

Early 2017, several months after we started recording and sharing our food journal online, I began attending a very intense exercise program. From January through May, I participated in a thrice-weekly, hour-long 6:15a spin class on campus at my work gym.

Usually, only seasoned exercise fanatics can get behind the notion of waking up at this hour consistently for months (or years on end). I considered myself in this group of dedicated fitness addicts and knew with certainty that I would lose thirty-plus pounds within these five months. I timed my still steady "good morning" group post to hit just as I parked the car and headed inside.

By not weighing in, I thought I was saving myself for a victorious, exuberant weigh-in when the class semester session ended. I told myself that not stepping on the scale might be the best approach to save myself from feelings of sadness and disappointment.

I did not realize that I already had a mechanism that eliminated the sadness associated with this issue. Checking in with friends and family in our group handled that part. At the end of the class, I had lost a whopping one pound. How is that for disappointment?

I share this story often to illustrate the folly of not weighing in. In contrast, after discovering intermittent fasting, I looked forward to daily morning weigh-ins, knowing I would see movement downward. I hypothesize that my spin class did not move the numbers because I was still eating breakfast, snack, lunch, dinner, weekend cheats, etc. Had I weighed in, I would have noticed sooner that my progress was not showing on the scale. Well, at least I had not gained, and we learn over time the value of that victory.

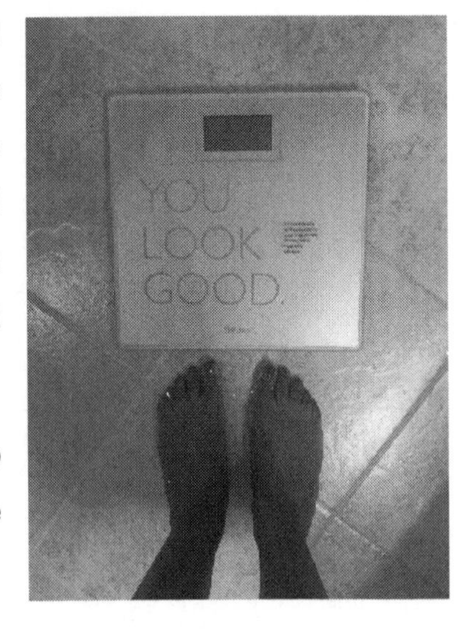

Buy a scale today if you do not own one. Do not be afraid.

A month of encouragement

1. There is no such thing as tomorrow, do it today

2. If working out were easy, everyone would have a six-pack

3. [It is] not worth it (It = the name of whatever offending food is staring you in the face at the moment, cookies, ice-cream, pizza, etc.)

4. Why work out later when you can work out now

5. [It] will be there after you reach your goal (It = the same or different offending food referred to above)

6. Never miss a Monday

7. That is not your food (when tempted by OPF, aka other people's food)

8. Nothing tastes as good as healthy feels

9. The scale is your friend

10. You cannot hide from the mirror

11. Eat that now, wear it later

12. Drink water first, eat that later (to ride out a craving)

13. Think it, say it, do it, share it (healthy meals and workouts start in your mind, as do cravings and plans to skip your workout)

14. Sugar is the devil

15. It is okay not to eat all of it

16. If you would not eat that in front of a roomful of people, do not eat it alone

17. If you cannot stop at one bite, do not even try one bite

18. Clothes too big or too loose feels better than clothes too small or too tight

19. No one can lose weight for you, but you

20. You are 100 % in control of every morsel of food that touches your lips

21. [Insert offending food item] is not your friend and does not care about you

22. Phone a friend instead

23. Push just a little bit harder

24. If you have even one thought about NOT quitting, go with THAT thought

25. You did not gain it overnight; you will not lose it overnight

26. If you can make it through the next 5 minutes, you can make it through to the endzone

27. Restart daily; every day is a new opportunity to get it right

28. You will never regret NOT eating that; you will most likely regret it if you DO

29. Ride it out until someone notices; the day is coming

30. If you had done what you were supposed to do this time last year, imagine how much further you would be. Do not repeat this next year

31. Early bird gets the workout worm

Conclusion

Congrats! You made it to the finish line of this glorious book if I am allowed to pat myself on the back. You may not be surprised to find that there is no conclusion to this story because we are all still learning. Never give up! It sounds cliché, but it is worth saying.

If you would like to reach me to discuss personalized one-on-one sessions, I am easy to find in all the usual places: on Clubhouse, Facebook, Instagram, TikTok, Twitter, YouTube.

www.3hourwindowdiet.com

www.8020journal.com

Acknowledgements

Thank you to the top dozen posters in *80/20 Journal*
without whom, none of this
would have been so much fun and worthwhile:
Annie, Bernard, Domenick, La Vona, Love, Melissa,
Monica, Nathan, Nichelle, Rick, Ronda, TK

Marta Saftescu: book cover art illustration

Renée and Katy, from Praise & Workout to 80/20 Journal:
your presence then and now blesses my whole soul

King Tone's revolutionarily powerful and enduring words :
"Numbers UP", "Group Force Dynamics", "No Sugary Snacks",
"Harness", "Queen Bee", "Generator", "Analytics"

Cheryl, Jackie B., Linda, Nicole, Tim, Wayne: family supporters

Julian, Kathy, Luna, Malaika, Melissa, Sarah, Stephen:
early adopters, posters, supporters and school chums

Jackie, Latrese, Sharon:
inspirational before and after results posters

Fasting Divas: Laquaia, Melissa, Vernise

Regularly engaging and encouraging:
Alex, Angela, Chiara, Elizabeth, Gail, Janice, Joelah,
Kim, Marisol, Mary, Rebecca, Shara, Vig

One-on-one coaching participation: Nora

Robin & Shannon: inspiring real life fitness trainers

Made in the USA
Middletown, DE
18 March 2021